The Nature I
The Amazonian Warrior
Workout

Written by:

Braeden Baade

Formatted by:

Damien Benoit-Ledoux

http://damienledoux.com/

http://www.NaturePhysiqueFitness.com

Braeden Baade

THE NATURE PHYSIQUE: THE AMAZONIAN WARRIOR WORKOUT
Copyright © 2017 Braeden Baade

To all the strong women out there and, as always, to all who endeavor to live a healthy life.

Table of Contents

Braeden Baade

Author's Note

If at any point, you feel that the following material fails to captivate, I'd like to give the option to immediately dive into the instructional portions of this book. I realize some readers may find some content to be irrelevant but I did feel an obligation to elaborate a bit on the origin of this book.

Disclaimer

All information and opinions expressed within this material are entirely my own and based upon my own personal perspective and experiences. I do not purport that this information is based on any accurate, current or valid scientific knowledge and as such *The Nature Physique: The Amazonian Warrior Workout* will not be liable for any losses, injuries or damages arising from its display or use. Please use your own discretion when exercising and consult your health-care provider if you feel any discomfort when performing any of the included exercises.

Your Free Book!

As a way of saying *thanks* for your purchase, I'm offering a free book to my readers.

This free book is attached at the end of The Nature Physique: The Amazonian Warrior Workout.

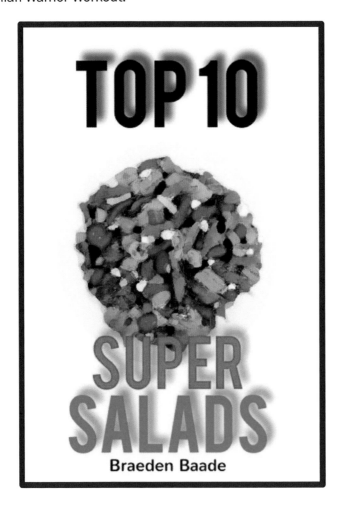

Foreword

Even though my premiere book *The Nature Physique* is intended to be utilized by all who read it, an idea dawned on me while writing it that I'd like to create a guide which specifically targets and enhances the female physique.

When working as a personal trainer in New York, it was a common occurrence when signing up a new female client for her to assure me that she most certainly didn't want a workout routine that would "bulk her up into the Hulk". I couldn't help but chuckle a bit before explaining to my new client that there is truly so much more that contributes to the objective of "bulking up" than just a mere 20-minute exercise routine, no matter what the routine consists of.

After the passing of a few weeks, it was always satisfying to see the client at ease when realizing that our tailored workout routine was delivering the results that she desired, as opposed to the potential "Hulk-like" appearance that was previously a concern.

There will never come a time when I recommend that dedicating a workout regimen to only a few select muscles is in any way beneficial for the human body; however, based on all of the input I received from my respected female clientele, it seemed advantageous to draft up a few customized routines. It was important for these routines to provide my clients with a sense of confidence and reassurance that they were targeting their most-desired muscles and at the same time assuring myself that they were receiving a healthy, full-body workout.

Braeden Baade

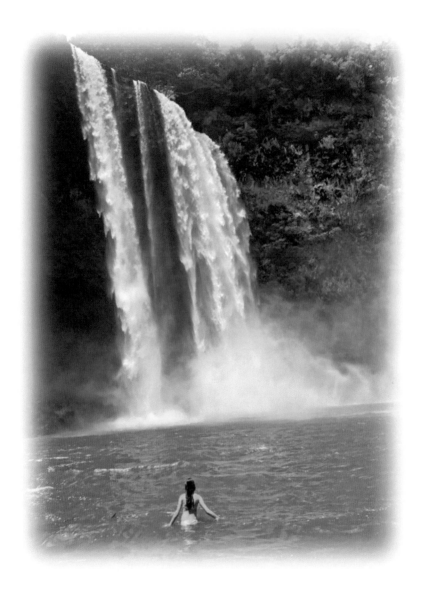

Required Materials

Resistance Bands are required to complete the following exercise routines. They can be purchased at most sporting goods stores, as well as from online retailers such as Amazon. I highly recommend you purchase a set that contains three different tensions so that you can efficiently increase the tension as your strength and endurance increases.

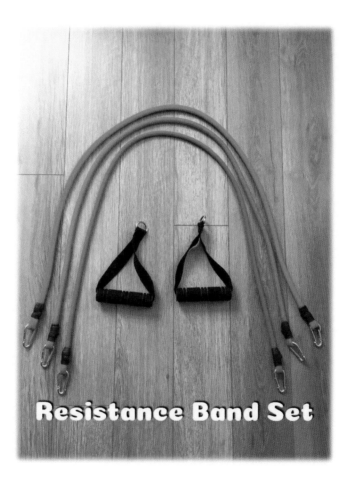

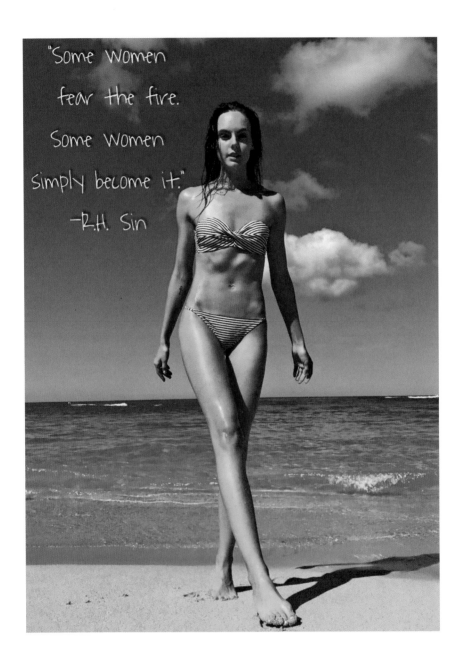

"Some Women fear the fire. Some Women simply become it."
—R.H. Sin

IMPORTANT TIPS

- It's extremely beneficial to first review the form of all included exercises before beginning the designated workout routine.

- The primary reason for including multiple routines is that muscles eventually adapt to the motion of any strenuous exercise. I'm not implying that any of the following exercises will become super easy for you, but a better analogy would be to say that muscles become "bored" after weeks upon weeks of the same motions. It's no secret that this can discourage your muscles from further progress; therefore, altering your routine every few weeks has been shown to be beneficial.

Braeden Baade

The Escape Portal:
A Technological Substitute for The Nature That We All Love

The Escape Portal series transports the viewer to an exotic location for an hour of audiovisuals from natural environments across the globe, which enables the viewer to digitally immerse themselves in nature.

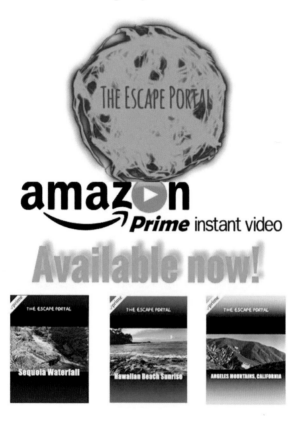

I made sure these videos were made FREE to watch for all Amazon Prime subscribers because I wanted my readers to have the next best thing for when they're unable to go outside to exercise. I will continue to expand the collection, so frequently check to see what's new! The *Escape Portals* can be viewed on smartphones, tablets, and computers.

Amazonian Warrior Novice Circuit

This first interval circuit targets various muscle groups to complete a full-body workout. I'd recommend performing it two to three times per week for at least four consecutive weeks before moving to the next routine.

This circuit includes the following exercises:

1) **Squat press** – 30 reps
Rest for 20 seconds

2) **Jump squats** – 10 reps
Rest for 20 seconds

3) **Knee push-ups** – 15 reps
Rest for 20 seconds

4) **Short bridge** – 30 reps
Rest for 20 seconds

5) **Resistance band row** – 30 reps
Reset for 20 seconds

6) **Stump dips** – 20 reps
Rest for 20 seconds

7) **Lying leg raise** – 15 reps
-Rest for 20 seconds, then the circuit.

- Have a stopwatch on hand (a smart phone works quite well).
- Repeat the circuit three times.
- Depending on your current fitness level, you may feel unable to reach the listed repetition amount; it's important to remember that that's perfectly acceptable. Do what you can and always do your best to push yourself!

Exercise #1: The Squat Press

This first exercise works both upper body and lower body muscles; primarily the quadriceps, glutes, hamstrings, and deltoids (shoulders).

- Begin by locating a flat, sturdy surface to stand.
- Position your feet so that they are shoulder-width apart and connect your palms in front of your chest (just as someone would when they're in prayer).
- Initiate the motion by lowering your glutes until they're nearly level with your knees. Now, as you smoothly rise, reach your hands toward the sky, forming an arrow-like shape. Take a slight pause, then lower your palms back to chest level.
- Repeat for 30 reps.
- Rest for 20 seconds.

The Squat Press

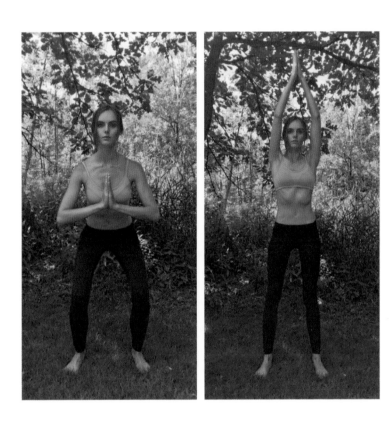

Exercise #2: The Jump Squat

Performing this exercise immediately after the squat press will be a bit tough but will work wonders for shocking your muscles into reaching new heights.

- Use the same flat, sturdy surface that you just used for the squat press exercise.
- Position your feet so that they're shoulder-width apart, and rest your hands loosely at your sides.
- Begin the motion by lowering your glutes until they are just above level with your knees, then quickly jump as high as you can while simultaneously reaching your hands for the sky. Make sure to give special attention to landing as softly on the ground as possible to avoid any potential injuries.
- Repeat for 10 reps.
- Rest for 20 seconds.

The Jump Squat

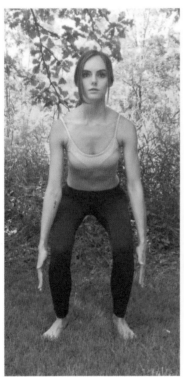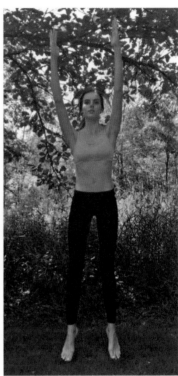

Exercise #3: The Knee Push-Up

This exercise targets your chest, shoulders, and triceps; it's a great time to perform this upper body exercise because I'm almost certain that your lower body will be begging for a short break by this point.

- Begin by locating a flat and sturdy surface.
- Get down on your knees and position your hands so that they are just a tad bit wider than shoulder-width. Position your knees so they're spread hip-width apart. Make sure to flex your abs as this will encourage good form.
- To initiate the motion, lower your body toward the ground until your elbows create a 90-degree angle, then push back up to the starting position.
- Repeat for 15 reps.
- Rest 20 seconds.

The Knee Push-Up

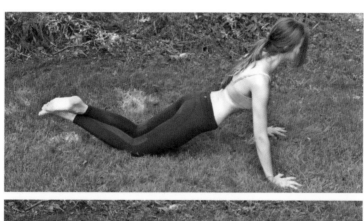

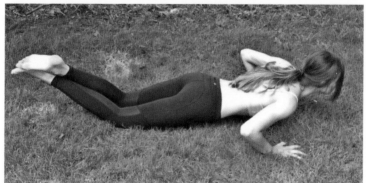

Exercise #4: The Short Bridge

This exercise is an excellent technique for increasing optimal glute and lower back strength. Fun fact: the gluteus maximus is the largest muscle in the human body!

- Begin by locating a flat, sturdy, and comfortable surface to lie on your back.
- Position your feet to create a 90-degree bend in the knees. Place your arms comfortably out to the sides.
- To initiate the motion, raise your pelvis in the air until it can't go any further. Remember to pause momentarily while squeezing your glutes before returning to the starting position.
- Repeat for 30 reps.
- Rest for 20 seconds.

The Short Bridge

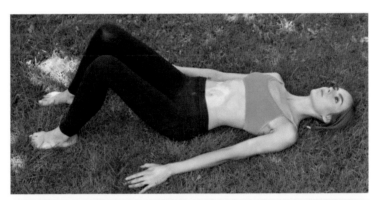

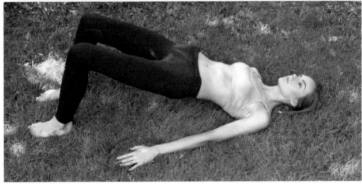

Exercise #5: The Resistance Band Standing Row

The resistance band standing row targets your biceps, as well as multiple regions of the back.

- Begin by locating a sturdy tree to anchor the center of the resistance band.
- Stand facing the tree with about four feet of space in between and anchor the band so that it's just below chest-level.
- To begin the motion, pull the handles inward until they nearly touch your chest and squeeze your back momentarily before gently returning to the starting position.
- Repeat for 30 reps.
- Rest for 20 seconds.

The Resistance Band Standing Row

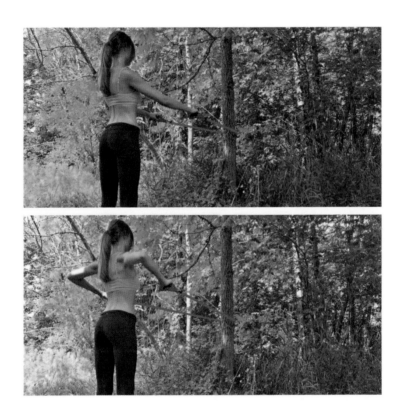

Exercise #6: The Stump Dip

This exercise is great for exhausting the triceps and increasing all-around definition throughout the upper arm.

- Begin by locating either a sturdy tree stump, park bench, or chair (if indoors).
- Stand with your back turned toward the rock, lower your body, anchor your hands on the edge, and bend your knees to about 90 degrees as if you were sitting in a chair.
- To begin the motion, slowly dip your body until your elbows are nearly bent to a 90-degree angle (as you shouldn't go any lower to avoid risking injury). Carefully push upward to the starting position.
- Repeat for 20 reps.
- Rest for 20 seconds.

The Stump Dip

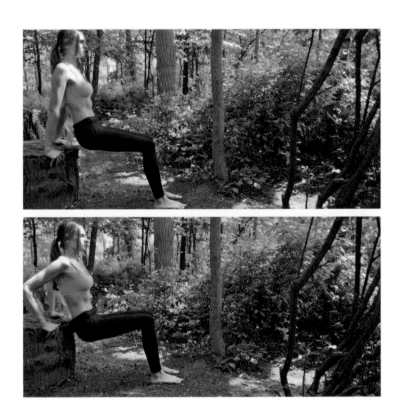

Exercise #7: The Lying Leg Raise

The lying leg raise is extremely effective when it comes to improving strength and definition within the lower abdominal muscles.

- Begin by locating a flat and comfortable surface to lie on.
- Lie down on your back with feet extended all the way forward. Place your arms at your sides and slide your hands (palms touching the ground) just underneath your glutes and keep them there for the duration of the exercise; this positioning is intended to help support the lower back.
- With both feet touching, raise your legs upward until a 90-degree angle is formed between your stomach and your quadriceps; take a slight pause before carefully lowering back down to the starting position.
- Repeat for 15 reps.

The Lying Leg Raise

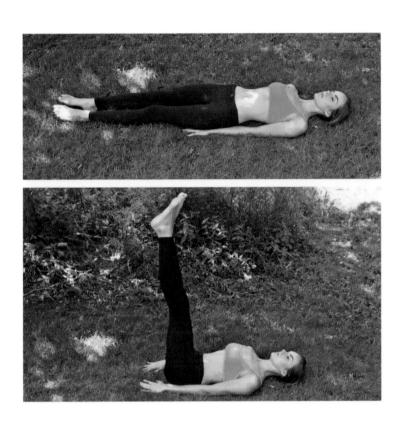

Braeden Baade

How Did You Like the First Circuit?

I'd like to take this moment to congratulate you on working through the novice circuit; you are now closer to uncovering your inner *nature physique* and I can't emphasize enough just how happy that makes me.

In order to reach more readers and help even more people just like you to reach their fitness goals, it would mean the world to me if you could quickly provide a rating and a short review at the book's Amazon.com page.

Also, if you're looking for a way to conveniently and effectively achieve a six-pack set of abs, I'd love for you to check out *The Nature Physique: Easy Breezy Abs*. This book is specially designed for busy individuals who don't often have the time or desire to go to the gym but are looking for some useful ab routines that can be done at home, on the road, or in nature!

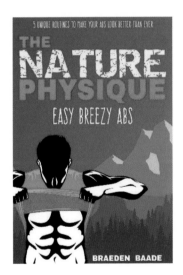

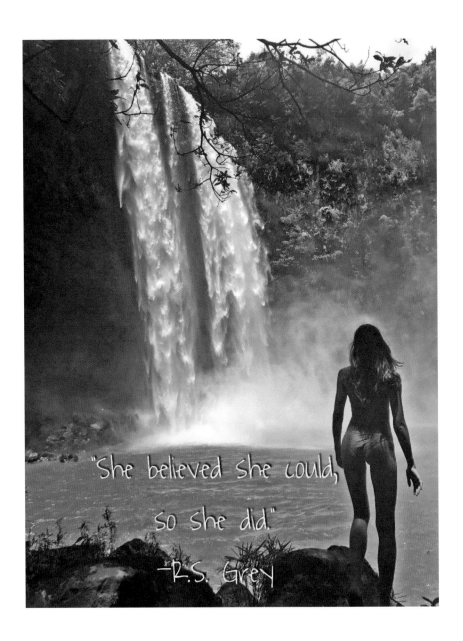

Amazonian Warrior Intermediate Circuit

Interval circuit #2 targets various muscle groups to complete a full-body workout. Upon completing an exercise, immediately proceed into the following exercise. I'd recommend performing this circuit two to three times per week with at least two days between.

This circuit includes the following exercises:
1) **Basic push-ups** – 10 reps
2) **Single leg squats** – 40 reps (20 each side)
3) **Chin ups** – 5 reps
4) **Calf raises**– 50 reps
5) **Resistance band overhead tricep extensions** – 30 reps
6) **Crisscrosses** – 30 reps
   -Rest for 60 seconds then repeat the circuit.

- Have a stopwatch on hand (a smart phone works quite well).
- Repeat the circuit three times.
- Depending on your current fitness level, you may feel unable to reach the listed repetition amount; it's important to remember that that's perfectly acceptable. Do what you can and always do your best to push yourself!

Exercise #1: The Basic Push-Up

This exercise targets your chest, shoulders, and triceps.

- Begin by locating a flat and sturdy surface.
- Get down on the ground and position your hands so that they are just a tad bit wider than shoulder-width. Position your feet so they're spread hip-width apart. Make sure to flex your abs as this will encourage good form.
- To initiate the motion, lower your body toward the ground until your elbows create a 90-degree angle, then push back up to the starting position.
- Repeat for 10 reps.

The Basic Push-Up

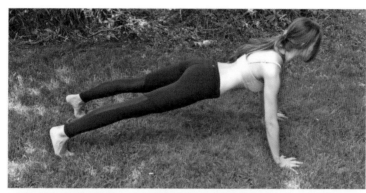

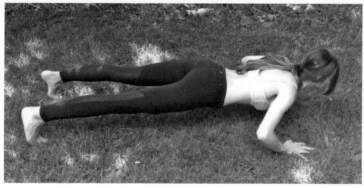

Exercise #2: Single Leg Squats

This next exercise focuses on strengthening and defining your quadriceps, hamstrings, and glutes. It is also exceptional for improving overall balance.

- Begin by locating a flat and sturdy surface to stand.
- With feet spread hip-width, gently rest your hands on your hips and leave them there for the duration of the exercise.
- To initiate the motion, raise your left foot off the ground and position it a bit behind your body. Now, just as you would with a basic squat, stick your butt out and bend your right knee as you carefully lower your body. Smoothly rise back up and repeat with the other leg.
- Repeat for 40 reps (20 each side).

Single Leg Squats

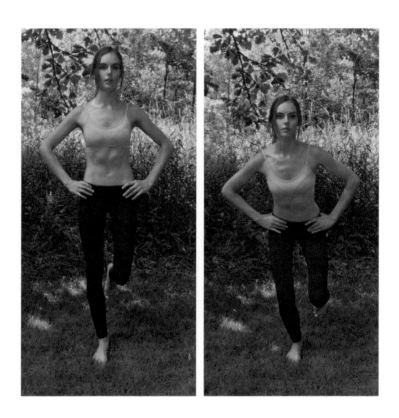

Exercise #3: The Chin Up

This exercise is a variation of the pull up and is highly effective for increasing strength, endurance, and definition within the upper back and bicep muscles.

- Begin by locating a sturdy tree branch that is within overhead reaching distance (if it's available, you can of course substitute with an actual pull up bar).
- To initiate the motion, reach for the branch with palms facing inward and elbows spread shoulder-width. Now, pull yourself up until your chin is just over the branch; hold for a slight pause while flexing your back muscles, then gently lower yourself to the starting position.
- Repeat for 5 reps.

The Chin Up

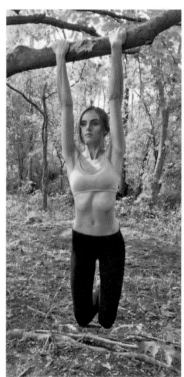 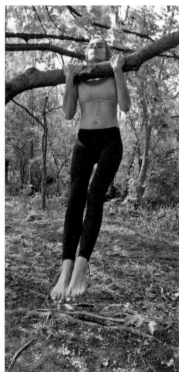

Exercise #4: The Calf Raise

This basic exercise focuses entirely on the calf muscles while also improving balance.

- Begin by locating a flat and sturdy surface to stand.
- Position your feet so that they're hip-width apart. Cross your arms over your chest and keep them there for the duration of the exercise.
- To initiate the motion, raise both of your heels off the ground as high as they can go, then softly return them to the ground.
- Repeat for 50 reps (or until you feel an intense burn).

The Calf Raise

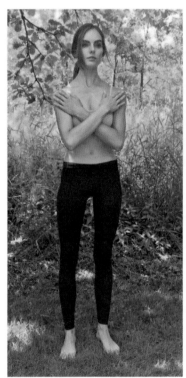 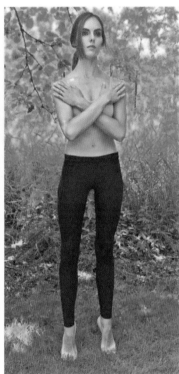

Exercise #5: The Resistance Band Overhead Tricep Extension

This exercise is extremely effective for carving and strengthening the upper arms; it will also boost your ability with all upper body pushing motions since the triceps are engaged in nearly every one of them.

- Begin by locating a sturdy object to sit on. Position your feet so that they're hip-width apart: place the middle of the resistance band under the souls of your feet. Ensure that there is an even amount of distribution of tension on both sides of the band.
- Grasp the handles behind your head and position your elbows so that they're pointing outward in front of you.
- To initiate the motion, push your forearms upward until they are aligned with your upper arms. Gently return to the starting position.
- Repeat for 30 reps.

The Resistance Band Overhead Tricep Extension

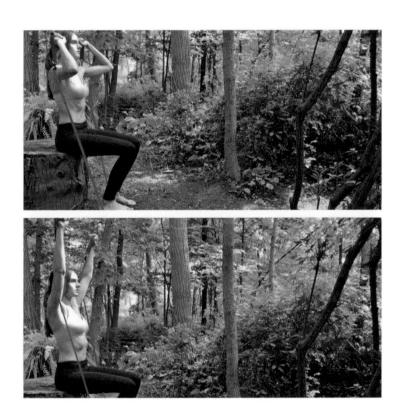

Exercise #6: The Crisscross

The crisscross is a highly effective exercise for increasing strength and endurance within the lower region of the abdominals.

- Begin by locating a flat and comfortable surface.
- Lie down on your back and extend your legs fully forward, feet should be shoulder-width apart, with heels only a few inches above ground. Place your arms at your sides with your hands tucked under your glutes for support.
- Initiate the motion by moving your feet inward and allowing them to cross over one another. Cross your right foot over your left foot, extend back outward, then cross your left foot over your right foot, extend back outward. Do not let your feet touch the ground for the duration of the exercise.
- Repeat for 30 reps.

The Crisscross

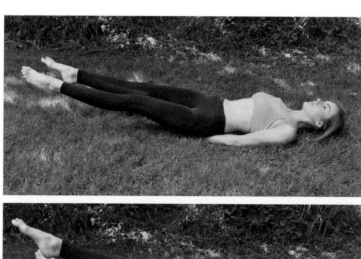

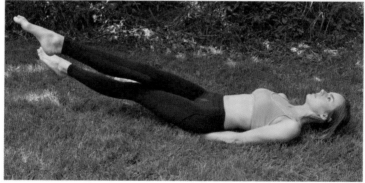

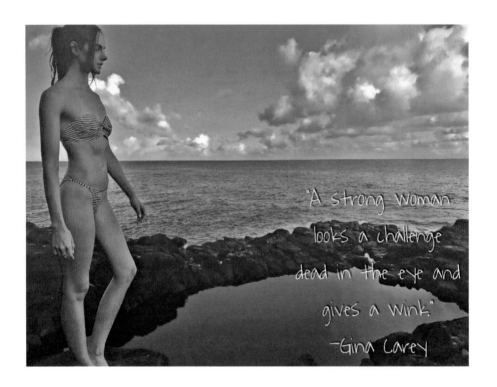

Amazonian Warrior Advanced Circuit

Interval circuit #3 is considerably more challenging than the previous circuits. I'd recommend performing this routine only if you are well conditioned.

This circuit includes the following exercises:
1) **Burpees** – 10 reps
2) **Resistance band front raises** – 30 reps
3) **Side kick squats** – 30 reps (15 each side)
4) **Basic crunches** – 30 reps
5) **Spider-man push-ups** – 10 reps
6) **Reverse grip resistance band lat pulldown** – 30 reps
7) **Jumping jacks** – 50 reps
-Rest for 2 minutes before repeating the circuit.

- Have a stopwatch on hand (a smart phone works quite well).
- Repeat the circuit three times.
- Depending on your current fitness level, you may feel unable to reach the listed repetition amount during the second and third rounds of the circuit; it's important to remember that that's perfectly acceptable. Do what you can and always do your best to push yourself!

Exercise #1: The Burpee

This first exercise of this circuit is quite a challenging one, hence why it's logical to perform it at the beginning while your endurance is at the maximum.

- Begin by locating a flat and sturdy surface to stand and position your feet so that they're hip-width apart.
- Initiate the motion by swiftly lowering into a squat position, place your palms on the ground, kick your feet backward into a push-up position, perform the push-up, quickly return to squat position, then jump up in the air as high as you can while reaching your hands for the sky.
  Repeat for 10 reps.

The Burpee

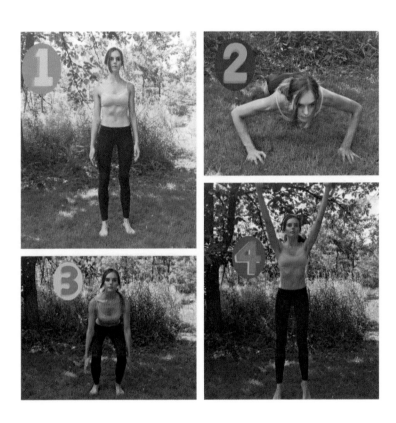

Exercise #2: The Resistance Band Front Raise

This next exercise focuses solely on developing definition and endurance within the deltoid muscles (shoulders); it is great for performing immediately after the previous burpees since the designated muscles will already be "pumped".

- Begin by locating a flat and sturdy spot on the ground.
- Position your feet so that they are spread hip-width apart. Place the center of the band underneath your feet while double-checking that there is an even amount of tension on both sides.
- To begin the motion, simultaneously lift both arms forward and upward until your hands are level with your shoulders. Maintain a slight bend within the elbows throughout the duration of the exercise.
- Repeat for 30 reps.

The Resistance Band Front Raise

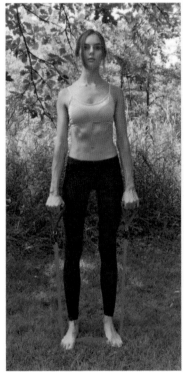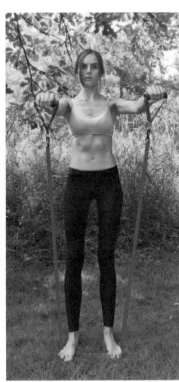

Exercise #3: The Side Kick Squat

This exercise is a unique spin on the basic squat; it will trigger the same, primary muscle groups but also serves as a method for improving balance.

- Begin by locating a flat and sturdy surface to stand.
- Spread your feet wider than you would with the basic squat, almost as if you were a sumo wrestler, and place your hands on your hips (or wherever feels most comfortable).
- To begin the motion, lower your body down until your glutes are about even with your knees. Then, quickly but smoothly rise while kicking your right leg outward to your right side. Bring your leg back in and repeat the motion but with your left leg.
- Repeat for 30 reps (15 each side).

The Side Kick Squat

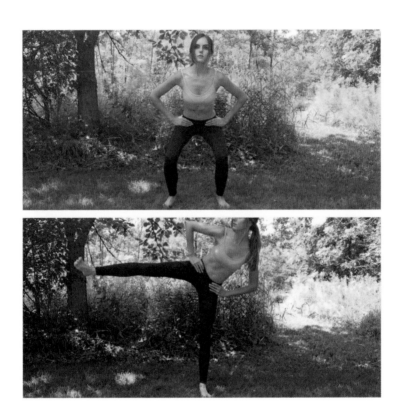

Exercise #4: The Basic Crunch

The basic crunch is one of the most common and most effective exercises for improving strength and increasing definition within the abdominal muscles.

- Begin by locating a flat and comfortable surface.
- Lie down on your back and position your knees so that the angle between your hamstrings and calves is about 90 degrees. Position your fingertips so that they're in contact with the back of your ears (maintain this placement of the finger tips without using your hands for support of the head). Hold your elbows out toward your sides while rounding them slightly inward.
- Initiate the motion by curling your chest upward (elevating the shoulder blades from the ground), as if attempting to connect your face to the sky, keeping your eyes focused straight up to the clouds or to the ceiling. Pause for a moment before gently returning to the starting position.
- Repeat for 30 reps.

The Basic Crunch

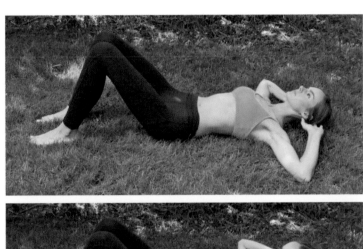

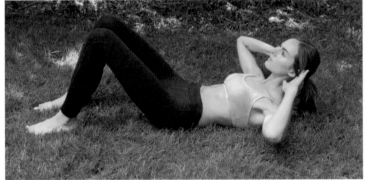

Exercise #5: The Spiderman Push-Up

This exercise is an advanced variation of the basic push-up; as usual, it targets the chest and triceps while also exhausting the core muscles. This one may take some practice before correct form becomes consistent.

- Begin by locating a flat and sturdy spot on the ground.
- Get down on your hands and feet; spread them a bit wider than shoulder-width as you would during a basic push-up.
- To initiate the motion, lower your chest to the ground while bringing your right leg in until your right knee nearly touches your right elbow. Extend your leg back to the starting position as you push your torso upward. Next, mirror this motion with your left leg.
- Repeat for 10 reps (5 each side).

The Spiderman Push-Up

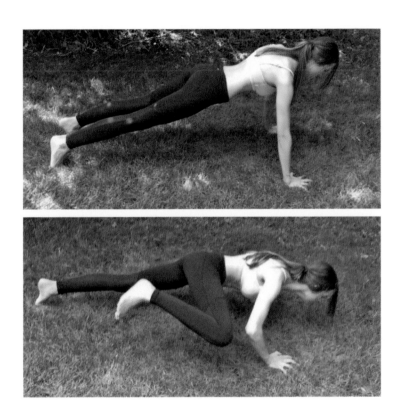

Exercise #6: The Reverse Grip Resistance Band Lat Pulldown

This exercise targets the muscles of the upper back, as well as the biceps; it's excellent for toning the arms and torso.

- Begin by locating a sturdy tree branch that is low enough to loop the resistance band a couple feet above your head.
- Position your hands so that they're shoulder-width apart, palms turned inward.
- To initiate the motion, pull down the handles until your elbows are aligned with your torso, take a slight pause, then gently return them to the starting position.
- Repeat for 30 reps.

The Reverse Grip Resistance Band Lat Pulldown

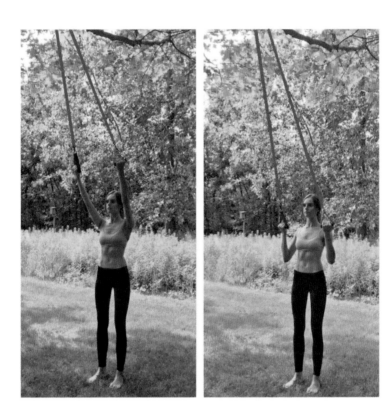

Exercise #7: Jumping Jacks

This common aerobic exercise is appropriate for performing at the end of this circuit; not only is it effective for conditioning the heart, it will help to keep you warmed up throughout your 2-minute break.

- Being by locating a flat and sturdy surface to stand.
- With great posture, position your feet together, arms loosely at your sides.
- To begin the motion, lightly hop off your feet, spreading them just beyond shoulder-width, while simultaneously raising your arms outward and upward until your hands nearly contact above your head. Return to the starting position. The key to this exercise is to be as light on your feet as you possibly can; in other words, no stomping!
- Repeat for 50 reps.

Jumping Jacks

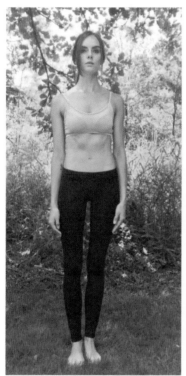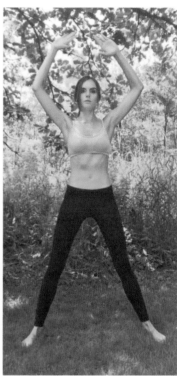

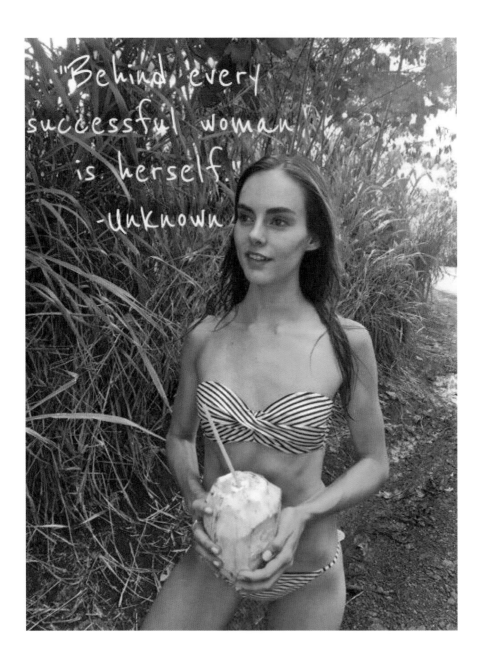

"Behind every successful woman is herself." -Unknown

Amazonian Warrior Master CIrcuit

The Amazonian Warrior Workout

Interval circuit #4 is considerably more challenging than the previous circuits. I'd recommend performing this routine only if you are well conditioned.

This circuit includes the following exercises:
1) **Resistance band single leg squats** – 40 reps (20 each side)
2) **Shoulder tap push-ups** – 10 reps
3) **Single leg calf raises** – 50 reps (25 each side)
4) **Resistance band bicep curls** – 30 reps
5) **Donkey kicks** – 70 reps (35 each side)
6) **Resistance band lateral raise** – 20 reps
7) **V-up crunches** – 15 reps
-Rest for 90 seconds, then repeat the circuit.

- Have a stopwatch on hand (a smart phone works quite well).
- Repeat the circuit three times.
- Depending on your current fitness level, you may feel unable to reach the listed repetition amount; it's important to remember that that's perfectly acceptable. Do what you can and always do your best to push yourself!

Exercise #1: The Resistance Band Single Leg Squat

The initial exercise of this circuit is an advanced variation of the single leg squat that was performed in a previous routine. It targets the quadriceps, hamstrings, and glutes.

- Begin by locating a flat and sturdy surface to stand.
- With the resistance band touching the ground, step on the middle of it with your right foot. Grasp the handles and position your hands so that they're leveled with your shoulders, palms facing outward; keep them there for the duration of the exercise.
- To initiate the motion, raise your left foot off the ground and position it a bit behind your body. Now, just as you would with a basic squat, stick your butt out and bend your right knee as you carefully lower your body. Smoothly rise back to the starting position and repeat with other leg.
- Repeat for 40 reps (20 each side).

The Resistance Band Single Leg Squat

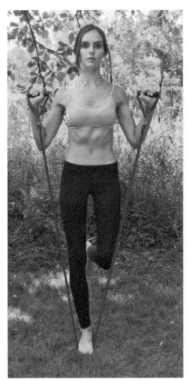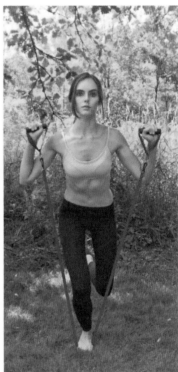

Exercise #2: The Shoulder Tap Push-Up

This exercise is an advanced version of the basic push-up; it works the muscles of the chest and triceps, and helps to improve balance.

- Begin by locating a flat and sturdy surface.
- Get down on the ground and position your hands so that they are just a touch wider than shoulder-width. Position your feet so they're spread hip-width apart. Make sure to flex your abs as this will encourage good form.
- To initiate the motion, lower your body toward the ground until your elbows create a 90-degree angle, then push back up to the starting position and tap your left shoulder with your right hand. Next, do the same motion but while tapping your right shoulder with your left hand.
- Repeat for 10 reps (5 each side).

The Shoulder Tap Push-Up

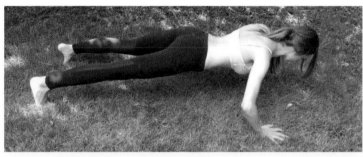

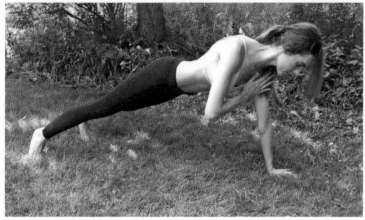

Exercise #3: The Single Leg Calf Raise

This exercise is highly effective for shaping and strengthening the lower leg muscles, as well as for improving balance.

- Begin by locating a flat and sturdy spot on the ground.
- Lightly rest your hands on your hips. Once you are comfortable, lift your left foot off the ground.
- To initiate the motion, raise your right heel upward as far as it can go and then gently lower it back to the ground. Next, mirror the motion with your left foot.
- Repeat for 50 reps (25 each side).

The Single Leg Calf Raise

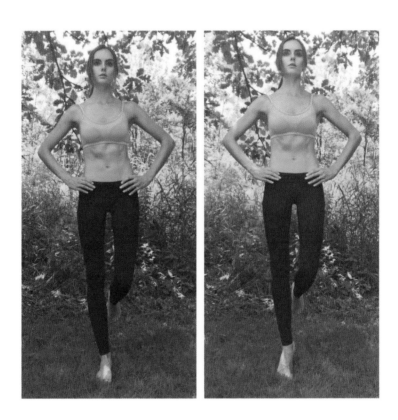

Exercise #4: The Resistance Band Bicep Curl

This basic exercise exhausts the bicep muscles and is incredibly effective for toning arms.

- Begin by locating a flat and sturdy surface to stand.
- Position your feet together and place the middle portion of the resistance band securely under your feet while ensuring that there is an even distribution of tension on both sides. Keep your elbows tucked in at your sides.
- Initiate the motion by simultaneously curling the resistance band handles upward until they nearly touch your shoulders. Then gently return to the starting position.
- Repeat for 30 reps.

The Resistance Band Bicep Curl

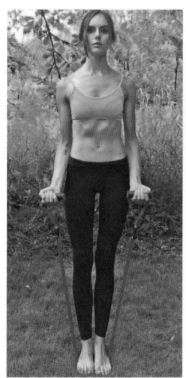 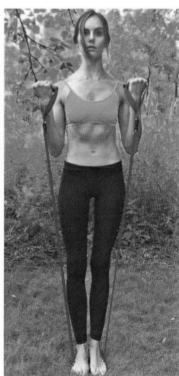

Exercise #5: The Donkey Kick

This exercise is incredibly effective for toning the hamstrings and glutes.

- Begin by locating a flat and supportive surface to get down on your hands and knees; make sure a 90-degree angle is formed between your hamstrings and calves, and that your hands are below your shoulders.
- Initiate the motion by flexing your right foot and lifting your right leg until your knee becomes parallel with your right hip. Then, gently return to the starting position with your right knee nearly touching the ground. Upon finishing the rep amount, repeat the motion with your left leg.
- Repeat for 70 reps (35 each side).

The Donkey Kick

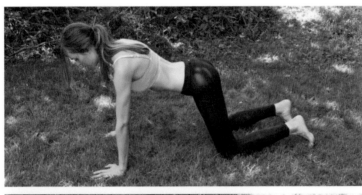

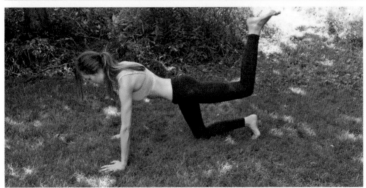

Exercise #6: The Resistance Band Lateral Raise

This exercise strengthens and tones the shoulders (without bulking them up); it will also help to increase definition within the arms.

- Begin by locating a flat and sturdy surface to stand.
- Position your feet together on the center of the resistance band and make sure there is an even amount of tension on each side. With palms facing inward toward your thighs, grasp the resistance band handles. Maintain a slight bend in your elbows throughout the exercise.
- To initiate the motion, raise your arms out from your sides until your hands are level with your shoulders. Briefly pause before gently lowering your arms to the starting position.
- Repeat for 20 reps.

The Resistance Band Lateral Raise

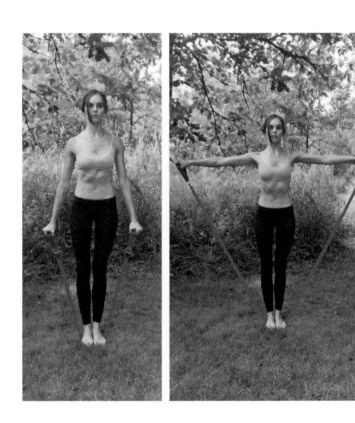

Exercise #7: The V-up Crunch

This final exercise of this circuit is super effective in terms of working both the upper and lower abdominal muscles within one smooth, controlled motion.

- Begin by locating a flat and comfortable surface to lie down.
- Lie on your back with your legs extended all the way forward, feet together. Extend your arms in the opposite direction, as if you'd be reaching for the sky if you were standing up.
- To initiate the motion, raise your legs (as you would in the lying leg raise exercise) and raise your arms until they nearly meet above your torso. Remember to also raise your torso off the ground in the same way you would perform a basic crunch. Lower back down to the starting position.
- Repeat for 15 reps.

The V-Up Crunch

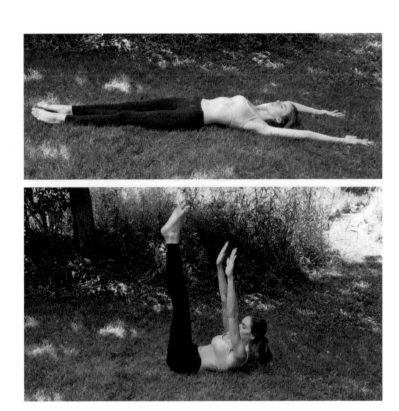

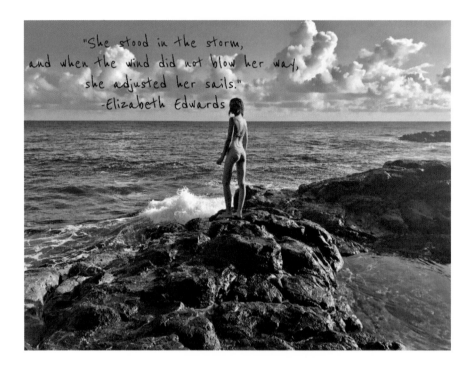

Conclusion

It is my hope that you will familiarize yourself with these routines and perform them on a consistent basis, thus helping you to see firsthand that eliminating fat and replacing it with lean muscle mass isn't nearly as complex as it is so often perceived.

Sculpting and strengthening those abdominal muscles is crucial for manifesting your inner *nature physique*!

Would You Like to Learn More?

You can learn quite a bit more on natural fitness within my other Kindle books. Guess what? I often run special promotions where I offer discounted (sometimes $0.99 or even FREE) books on Amazon.

A great way to find out about these offerings is to subscribe to my email list.

For a variety of full body workouts, check out *The Nature Physique* on Amazon.com.

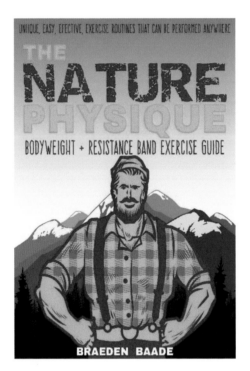

Nature Physique Fitness on YouTube

YouTube is another outlet I use to reach my readers. The Nature Physique Fitness channel is comprised of specific exercise tips, along with candid footage of my camping adventures and my admiration for the great outdoors. It would be incredibly appreciated if you could click the "subscribe" button; it's 100% FREE to do so.

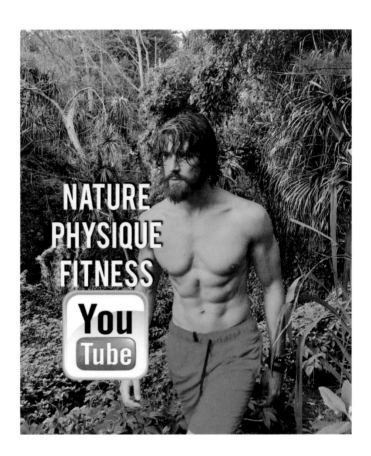

Did You Enjoy The Nature Physique: The Amazonian Warrior Workout?

Before you continue your fitness journey, I'd very much like to say "thank you" for downloading this guide. I'm aware that you had an endless variety of exercise books to select from, but you took a chance on my teachings.

At this point, I'd like to ask you for a *tiny* favor- could you submit a review on this book's Amazon page? Your feedback will aid me as I continue to create Kindle books that you, as well as others, can benefit from. If you happened to find A LOT of value within the content, be sure to let me know by shooting an email to braeden.baade@gmail.com :)

Last, but not least, feel free to visit:
http://www.NaturePhysiqueFitness.com from time to time, where you'll find new information on how to further improve your health and physique.

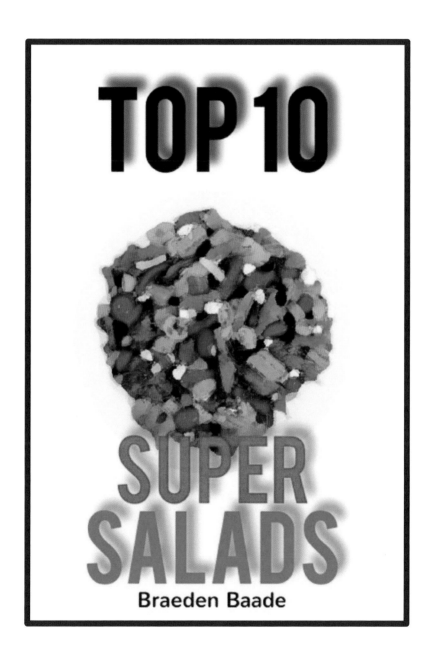

Top 10
SUPER SALADS

Written by:

Braeden Baade

Formatted by:

Damien Benoit-Ledoux

http://www.NaturePhysiqueFitness.com

TOP 10 SUPER SALADS

Copyright © 2017 Braeden Baade

All information and opinions expressed in *Top 10 Super Salads* are entirely the Author's and are based upon his own personal perspective and experiences. He does not purport the information presented in this book is based on any accurate, current or valid scientific knowledge and as such *Top 10 Super Salads* will not be liable for any losses, injuries or damages arising from its display or use. Please use your own discretion when consuming food products. As always, check with your doctor before beginning a new dietary regimen.

Introduction

Throughout the years, I've been frequently asked what I prefer to eat for breakfast, lunch, and dinner when the intention is to become/remain lean and fit. The truth is that the answer varies quite a bit. However, I do usually make sure to include at least a side salad with most afternoon and evening meals.

It goes without saying that salads are one the best techniques for combining a variety of nourishing ingredients into a single healthy and cost-effective dish. As with many other meals, finding the necessary ingredients that will compliment one-another can sometimes be challenging and tedious. Allow me to make this easy for you!

Feel free to experiment with the following recipes in order to match your taste; my hope is that you'll be pleasantly surprised by how delicious some of these salads can be.

Lemon Herb Chicken Salad

*This recipe serves 2

Dressing
- 2 tablespoons olive oil
- ¼ cup lemon juice
- 2 tablespoons water
- 2 tablespoons vinegar
- Chopped parsley
- 2 teaspoons dried basil
- 2 teaspoons minced garlic
- 1 teaspoon dried oregano
- 1 teaspoon salt
- Cracked pepper

Salad
- 2 grilled/broiled chicken breasts
- 2 cups lettuce
- 1 cup diced cucumber
- 1 diced tomato
- ½ diced onion
- 1 sliced avocado
- 1/3 cup sliced black olives

Salmon Caesar Salad

*This recipe serves 2

Dressing
- 2 tablespoons reduced fat mayo
- 3 tablespoons plain Greek yogurt
- 1 tablespoon olive oil
- 1 clove crushed garlic
- 1 chopped anchovy fillet
- 1 tablespoon lemon juice
- 1 tablespoon parmesan cheese
- Cracked pepper to taste

Salad
- 2 fresh salmon filets
- 1 tablespoon garlic powder
- 2 teaspoons lemon juice
- 2 poached eggs
- 1 cup lettuce
- 1 cup spinach
- 1 sliced avocado
- ½ cup shaved parmesan cheese

Kale and Brussels Sprouts Salad

*This recipe serves 2

Dressing
- ¼ cup tahini
- 2 tablespoons white wine vinegar
- 2 teaspoons raw maple syrup
- 2 teaspoons white miso
- Pinch of red pepper flakes
- ¼ cup water

Salad
- 1 bunch kale
- 2 handfuls brussels sprouts
- 3 tablespoons sliced almonds
- ¼ cup shaved parmesan cheese
- Pinch of sea salt

Honey Mustard Chicken Salad

*This recipe serves 4

Dressing
- ½ cup honey
- 3 tablespoons organic mustard
- 2 tablespoons olive oil
- 1 teaspoon minced garlic
- Pinch of salt

Salad
- 4 grilled/broiled chicken breasts
- 2 cups spinach
- 2 cups lettuce
- 1 cup sliced cherry tomatoes
- 1 sliced avocado
- ¼ cup corn kernels
- ¼ cup diced onion

Garlic Shrimp Caesar Salad

*This recipe serves 2

Dressing
- ¼ cup plain Greek yogurt
- 1 tablespoon reduced fat mayo
- ½ tablespoon olive oil
- 1 teaspoon minced garlic
- 1 tablespoon lemon juice
- 1 ½ tablespoon parmesan cheese
- Cracked pepper to taste

Salad
- 1 pound grilled shrimp
- Fresh squeezed lemon juice
- 1 tablespoon minced garlic
- 1 poached egg
- 2 cups spinach
- 2 cups lettuce
- 1 sliced avocado

Chickpea Avocado Salad

*This recipe serves 2

Dressing
- 2 tablespoons olive oil
- 1 tablespoon vinegar

Salad
- 2 cups spinach
- 2 cups lettuce
- 1 can rinsed chickpeas
- 1 cup sliced cherry tomatoes
- ½ cup reduced fat feta cheese
- 2 sliced avocados
- Cracked pepper to taste

Chipotle Carnitas Salad

*This recipe serves 4

Dressing
- ¼ cup olive oil
- ¼ cup pure lime juice
- 2 teaspoons minced garlic
- 1 teaspoon honey
- 1 finely chopped chili pepper
- ¼ cup chopped cilantro
- 1 teaspoon cumin
- Cracked pepper to taste

Salad
- Pulled pork
- ½ cup canned corn
- ½ sliced bell pepper
- 1 sliced Poblano pepper
- 3 cups lettuce
- 2 cups spinach
- 2 sliced avocados
- 1 cup red rice

Tropical Spinach Salad

*This recipe serves 1

Salad
- 3 cups baby spinach
- 1/3 cup chopped strawberries
- 1/3 cup chopped pineapple
- ½ sliced avocado
- 1/8 cup sliced red onion
- Shaved parmesan

Blackened Shrimp Salad

*This recipe serves 2

Dressing
- 1/3 cup Greek yogurt
- 1 teaspoon lemon pepper
- 1 teaspoon lemon juice
- 2 tablespoons olive oil

Salad
- 500g grilled shrimp
- 2 cloves minced garlic
- 1 teaspoon thyme
- 1 teaspoon sea salt
- 1 teaspoon cracked pepper
- 2 teaspoons cayenne pepper
- 2 teaspoons sweet paprika
- 2 bunches sliced asparagus
- 1 teaspoon olive oil

Lemon Parsley Bean Salad

*This recipe serves 6

Salad

- 2 cans rinsed red kidney beans
- 1 can rinsed chickpeas
- 1 diced red onion
- 2 sliced stalks celery
- 1 chopped tomato
- 1 diced cucumber
- ¾ cup chopped parsley
- 2 tablespoons chopped mint
- ¼ cup olive oil
- ¼ cup lemon juice
- 3 cloves minced garlic
- Pinch of sea salt
- Pinch red pepper flakes

Conclusion

I hope you feel inspired to consume a few (or more) of these tasty, healthy salads on a regular basis; they can be enjoyed at any time!

On another note, if you're often in search of new ways to challenge your body and improve your physique, I'd be honored if you would give my original book *The Nature Physique* a read. This book consists entirely of full-body resistance band and bodyweight training; the best part is that all of the workouts can be performed in under 20 minutes, at home... or in nature :)

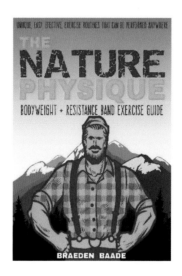

Did You Enjoy Top 10 Super Salads?

Before you continue your fitness journey, I'd very much like to say "thank you" for downloading this guide.

I'm aware you had an endless variety of health and fitness books to select from, but you took a chance on my teachings.

Therefore, some huge thanks for reading this guide and for sticking with it all the way to the last page.

At this point, I'd like to ask you for a *tiny* favor; it would mean the world to me if you could leave a review on the Amazon.com page for the book you purchased.

Your feedback will aid me as I continue to create products that you, as well as others, can benefit from. If you happened to find A LOT of value within the content, be sure to let me know :)

Last, but not least, feel free to visit: www.NaturePhysiqueFitness.com from time to time, where you'll find new information on how to further improve your health and physique.

19825808R00059

Printed in Poland
by Amazon Fulfillment
Poland Sp. z o.o., Wrocław